This book is dedicated to all of the families and patients out there who are dealing with dysautonomia or another invisible illness. May you be kind, feel loved, be supportive and help your family member live their best life. They are struggling and truly need the support and belief from their support network. It's a lonely battle at times, especially when doctors and other specialists do not believe you and what your family/friend is facing daily.

ISBN: 9798880278398

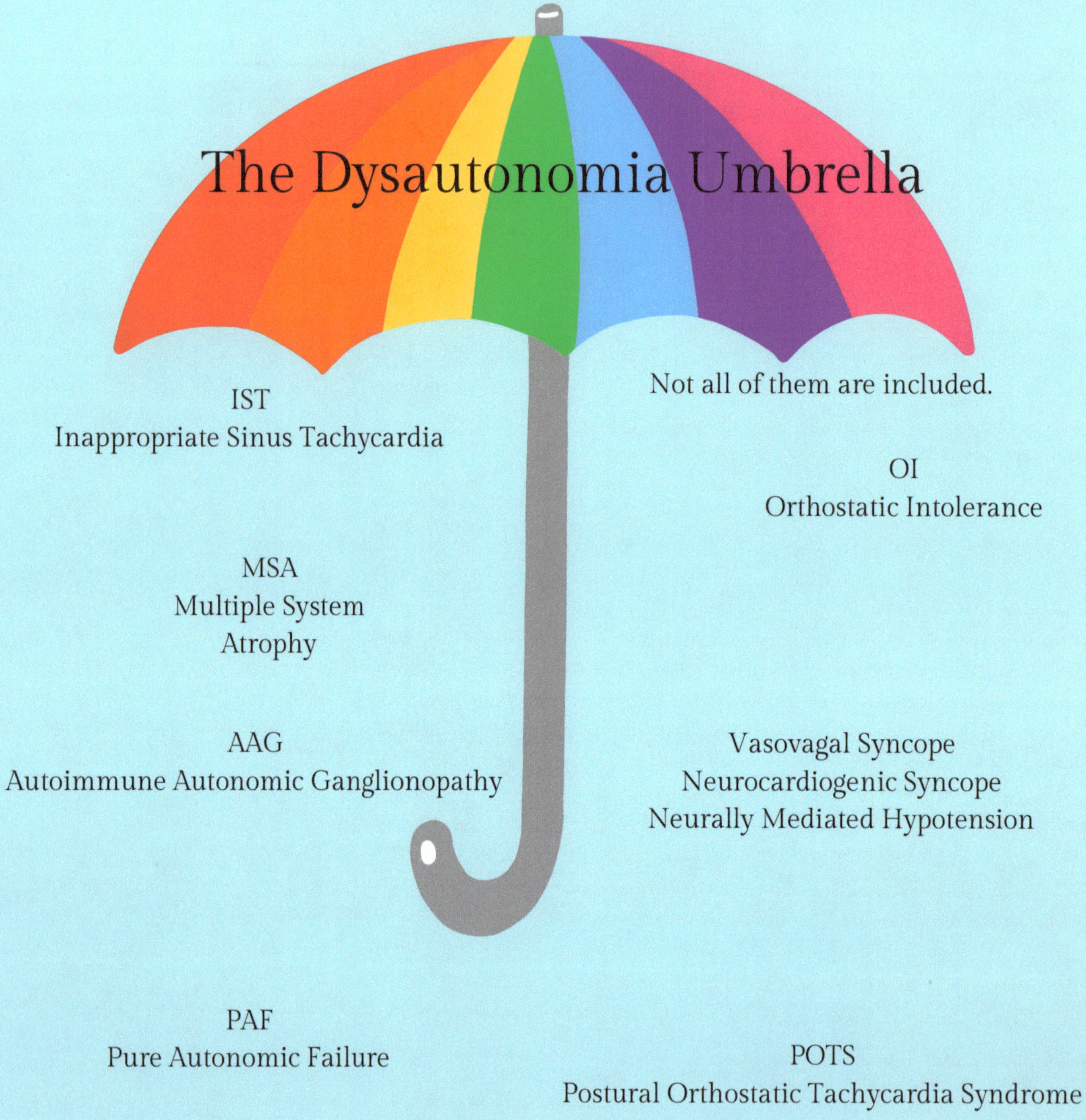
The Dysautonomia Umbrella
Not all of them are included.
IST
Inappropriate Sinus Tachycardia
OI
Orthostatic Intolerance
MSA
Multiple System
Atrophy
AAG
Autoimmune Autonomic Ganglionopathy
Vasovagal Syncope
Neurocardiogenic Syncope
Neurally Mediated Hypotension
PAF
Pure Autonomic Failure
POTS
Postural Orthostatic Tachycardia Syndrome

What is Dysautonomia?
This is an umbrella term that refers to any disorder of the ANS or autonomic nervous system.

Your body is an amazing machine. There are many functions of your body that just do things on their own without you even thinking about them.

These are "automatic" things such as breathing, heart rate, digestion, blood pressure regulation, your temperature regulation, how much you sweat or don't, sexual function, digestive, kidney and liver function, pupil dilation and constriction.

Recent medical advances and research have improved our understanding of dysautonomia, following long covid patients being diagnosed. It has taken some individuals years to have their physicians or family members truly believe them. The reason is because many have focused on their family or friend is making it up in their head and spiraling out of control or they are just having a panic attack and from the doctor that doesn't understand it, they just throw anxiety meds your way but do not address the passing out issues or other issues present.

Many patients have been told that it is all in their heads.

According to Dysautonomia International, over 70 million people have and live with a form of dysautonomia.

It can take up to seven years or longer to get a formal medical diagnosis, however, this is becoming shorter as more awareness is being brought to this illness.

It also is misunderstood as it can range from mild to extremely disabling and unfortunately death has been known to occur.

Treatments continue to be researched; however, it is not a one size fits all approach.
Some individuals can improve and do, but others will get worse.
Doctors do not have magic crystal balls that predict the long term outcomes and impacts of symptoms on an individual basis.

There are primary and secondary dysautonomia types to be aware of:
Primary- this condition can spontaneously happen without any other underlying condition.
Secondary- dysautonomia is related to another condition.

Primary dysautonomia is inherited and is called familial dysautonomia. There are three main reasons an individual would be diagnosed:

Having a family member with dysautonomia
Having a heritage of Eastern European descent
Your heritage might be the Ashkenazi form of Judaism.

Don't worry, just because you might be one of the above, does not mean that you will develop dysautonomia.

Some of the more common conditions associated with secondary dysautonomia are: traumatic brain injury, small fiber neuropathy, spinal cord injury, primary focal hyperhidrosis, rheumatoid arthritis, Sjogren's syndrome, vasovagal syncope, type 2 diabetes, Wernicke-Korsakoff syndrome, Sneddon Syndrome, toxins, molds, poisons, heavy metals, Parkinson's disease, orthostatic hypotension, multiple system atrophy, multiple sclerosis and more. When your autonomic nervous system is dysregulated, you can then develop dysautonomia as the co-existing condition.

Dysautonomia Symptoms:

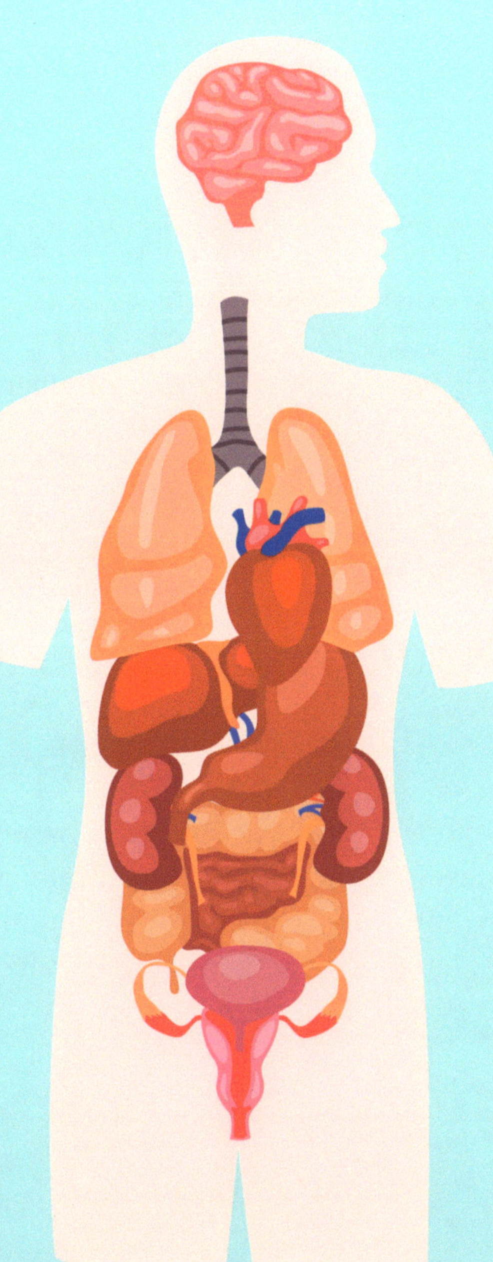

How can you best support your family member with dysautonomia or other chronic medical conditions?

First and foremost, believe them.
Do you think they want to be lying in bed all day or on a couch not participating in societal activities?

One of the hardest things is when patients do not feel heard.
This can cause increased anxiety.

Anxiety then worsens how a person can feel regardless of if they have dysautonomia or not.

There have been children and parents that have disowned their family members because they haven't taken the time to understand what their family member is going through.

The best thing you can do is: Listen, support, and encourage.

This journey is a long one.

Patients can often go several months between appointments.
With the short-staffed medical situation currently in the world, physicians, and other health practitioners that are knowledgeable about dysautonomia are in high demand and very few can you get into immediately. There are extensive wait lists. Doctors and other medical staff don't always fully understand exactly the "Why" behind Dysautonomia either.

If you are lucky as a patient, it could be from an autoimmune condition that co-exists that is caught early on. Otherwise, as anything, you treat the symptoms.

Some of the underlying conditions are mast cell activation syndrome or mast cell activation disease, Ehlers-Danlos Syndromes, Parkinson's disease, Sjogren's Disease, Diabetes, viruses, post-concussion syndrome and Chiari malformation.

Exercise is a huge part of the healing process; however, some patients have the hardest time due to fear of passing out, during the thing that is supposed to help them.

Encourage them. Take their hand, take a walk, swim next to them, be an encourager.

Go to doctor's visits with your friend or family also, hear how you can be of support.

Can you help and research on social media pages or other web pages available?

If they are having a "down" day, can you have groceries delivered, a meal provided or even to go sit with them and make them feel heard and seen.

Patient's, make sure you are also advocating for your needs as well in a healthy and respectful way. Have you told them how migraines can affect you and how they can help you during an episode?

Do you need your family/friend to whisper when you are having a headache, do you need a fan because you are sweating so much, do you need an extra blanket?

Remember, people are not mind readers and we all need to COMMUNICATE with each other in order to feel heard and supported.

<u>Specialist that can help support you:</u>

There are many specialists out there that can support you or your friend or family on their journey. However, as I mentioned previously, it can take a long time to get into someone that is truly knowledgeable about Dysautonomia.

In the area of pediatrics, it truly is much harder than in adults, to find specialists as well as running tests on kids.

Families have to travel at times hundreds of miles from home in order to go to an autonomic center or a
lab that can perform the necessary tests. These can take days to perform.

If there are siblings in the family, this can take a toll on them as well, as they are left behind often with a family member.

Other specialists out there are: cardiologists, neurologists, immunologists, rheumatology, psychiatry, dermatology, occupational therapy, aquatic therapy, physical therapy, speech therapy and your general practitioner. This of course is not the entire list, but it is a great start.

Start a journal immediately! That was one of the best pieces of advice!

Write down your symptoms, were you not able to get out of the bed, did you have a bowel or bladder accident? Did you have a headache and on a scale of 1-10 what was it?

Unfortunately, when you go to the emergency room, unless you are having a heart attack, and you have a
doctor that knows about dysautonomia, you will not be understood.

The frustration is real, but you are NOT ALONE.

Have a personal emergency action plan in place with a family member or friend. Have rescue meds in place that help you.

Before you pass out or are in pre-syncope, review strategies with your family and include helpful ways or strategies and other important information such as how to help you to the floor and what to do when you get there.

When you are getting out of bed in the morning, what are some ways they can help make your day better if you need it?

Dysautonomia can be very scary. Especially for those that do not understand what you are going through.

Remember that this disorder acts differently for each person. This means that even professionals need to know YOUR dysautonomia, to best help you.

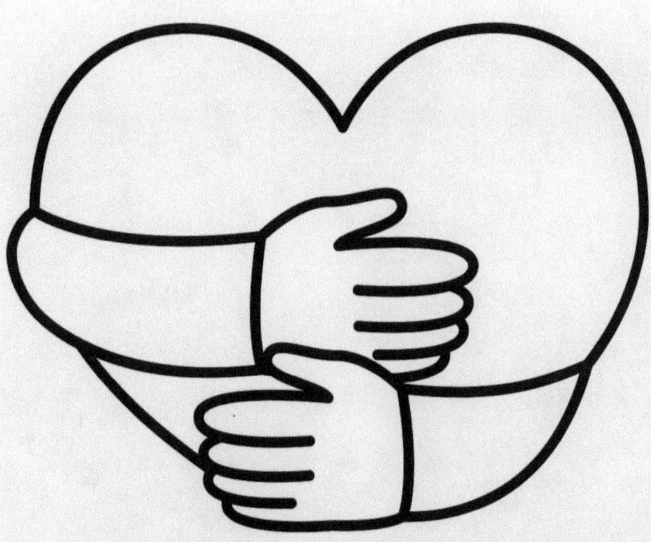

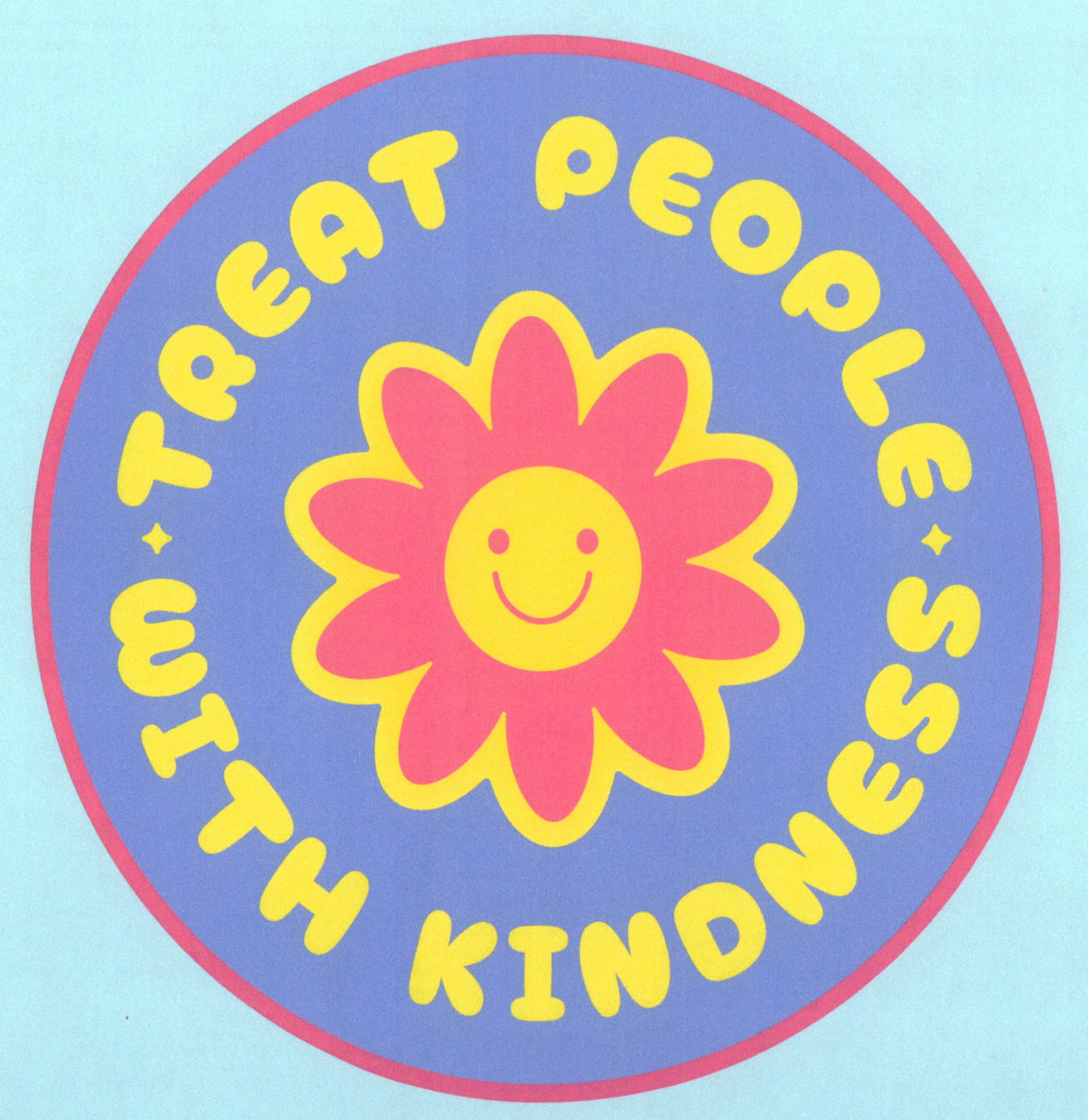

TREAT PEOPLE
WITH KINDNESS

<u>Employers and Their Role in Supporting Individuals with Dysautonomia</u>

Occupational therapist, can assist clients and others facing challenges with daily tasks, particularly in the realm of dysautonomia, where occupational therapy is often overlooked.

In the workplace:
For individuals with dysautonomia, especially those with POTS or OI who struggle with prolonged standing, workplace adjustments must be considered.

Refer to the American with Disabilities Act of 1990 to understand your rights.
It is essential to provide medical documentation of the condition, and always consult your physician to determine any limitations you may have.

Things to consider: Do you need to re-think how you work? Could you benefit from a job coach or speaking to HR about modifications and accommodations that they can provide you? Do you need to consider a different career path that allows you to work from home?

There are many possibilities to being able to live life and continue to be social!

So many people get stuck in a rut due to loneliness of this isolating illness, especially those that do not have a good social support network available to them.

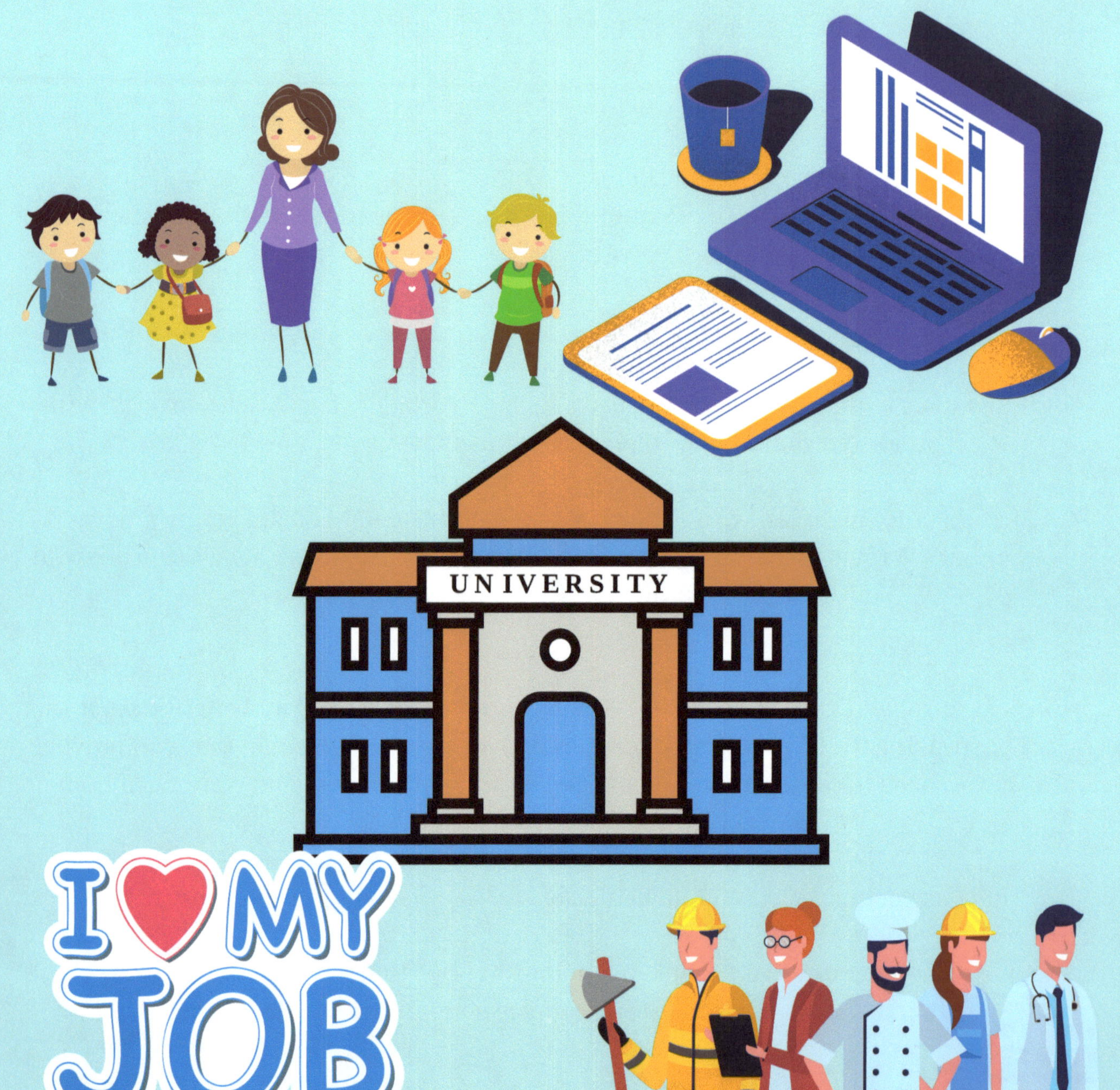

UNIVERSITY
I ❤ MY JOB

Educational Institutions (K-12 and College) and Their Supportive Role

These students can also suffer from anxiety. Just thinking about going to school and, having to use all of their spoons available to them is exhausting and scary.

Students may be thinking: What if I pass out while getting up from their desk? What if I have a bowel or bladder accident at school?

These are things you might not be thinking about, but they are. Will today be the day I can't play in physical education and their cheeks and ears are turning red? Will kids are making fun of them?

Do they need access to the school counselor or to the school psychologist?

Could they use a mentor/advisor that could help them and advocate to other teachers for the patients/young adults?

In college, do they need to have access to the disabilities center? What do they do if they can't make it to class one day? Plans need to be made and patients need to be involved in the decision-making process, but they can't do it alone.

This is where a parent comes in. Help your high school senior advocate for their needs for their next year in college. Modeling how to be an advocate and writing down any pertinent information is invaluable.

Help them find programs/schools that will help them feel successful.
ADVOCATE- ADVOCATE- ADVOCATE

There are many accommodations and modifications that can be put into place. The internet has reference tools including dysautonomia groups that have websites. They have so many great resources that have already been written! They make it easy to follow!

The Dysautonomia Journal is a great place to have all of your tools in your toolbox for information needs!

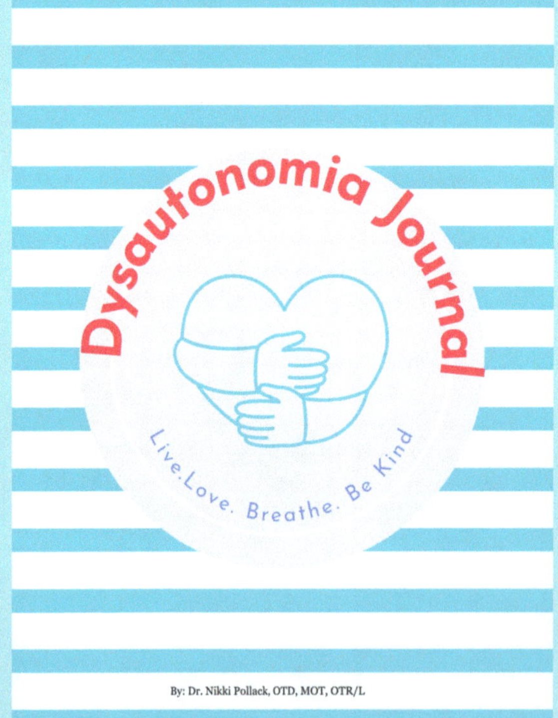

The Spoon Theory

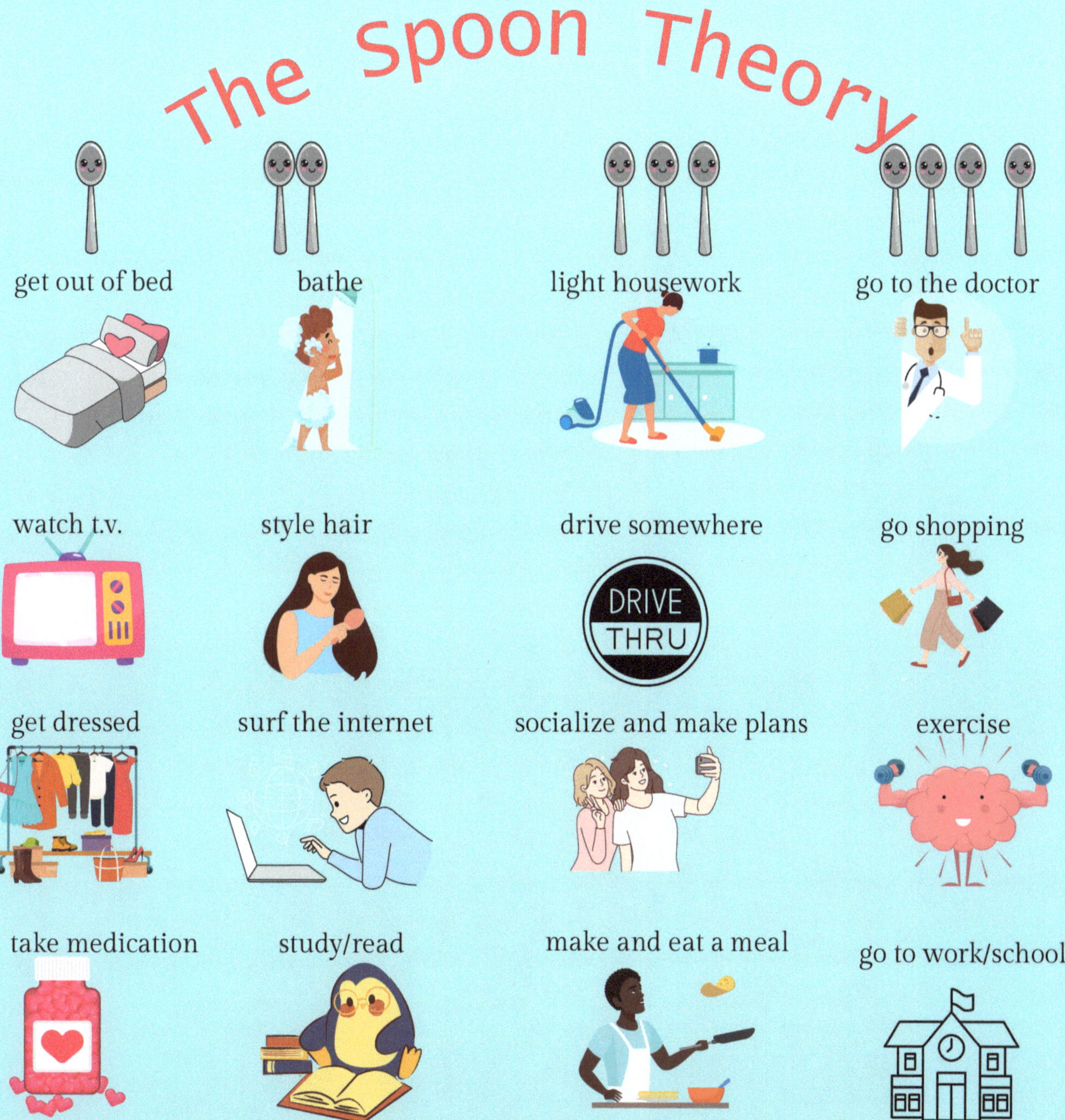

The Spoon Theory was created by Christine Miserandino at www.butyoudontlooksick.com

The Spoon Theory

For individuals with invisible chronic illnesses, chronic pain, and other disabilities the spoon theory allows individuals to have a visual that explains how much they can truly take either physically or mentally. This gives patients alternative ways to show others their energy level and exactly how each task of their activities of daily living can be impacted both physically and mentally.

You start with 12 spoons per day, you get to choose how to use them.

When completing activities of daily living such as showering, getting dressed, brushing your teeth, and most of us do not have to think about how much energy we have to put into them. For individuals with dysautonomia, these activities can be exhausting.

Have you ever been so tired from a night out at a party and you either had too many libations or you just had so much fun and stayed out too late?

This is the feeling that some of individuals with dysautonomia and other co-existing conditions face daily. It is critical to have medications or other tools in their toolbox to help them get through their day.

This theory provides a great visual, especially for younger kids that need help with explaining it to their families or friends.

This tool can also be useful for adults as well that have a difficult time with family/friends that don't quite understand why their energy is non-existent at times.

When kids want to go to a birthday party or a play date, they might need to rest and have more downtime than normal before the event. An adult or teenager, might need to rest longer in order to make it out that night, and even then, they might be so fatigued mentally or physically that they just can't make it. It's amazingly easy to judge another's life, until you have walked in their shoes.

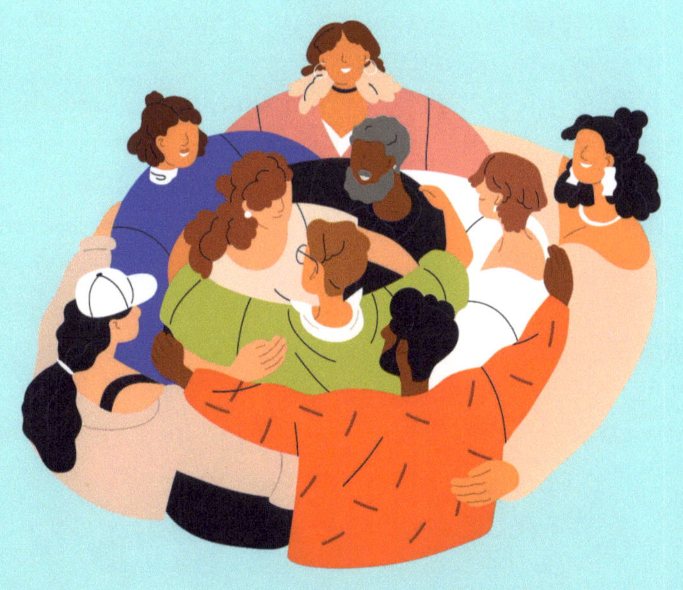
#BeKind

<u>Chronic Illness and Anxiety and Depression</u>

You don't feel well, you want to be heard and seen by people. If you are a caregiver, you are frustrated as you think the individual could do more than what they are, or they are making it up for attention.

There are different symptoms that someone with dysautonomia might be feeling, just as we looked at in the beginning of the book. Someone with POTS might be having shortness of breath, pain in their chest,

Anxiety does not cause dysautonomia, but dysautonomia can cause anxiety and depression.

Individuals with EDS or other connective tissue syndromes might struggle as well with complaints of headache, dizziness, tachycardia, chest pain, presyncope, gastrointestinal distress and more.

A lot of diagnoses overlap, so it is hard to determine which came first to a physician that has never met you. A lot like dementia, dysautonomia can start slowly in the early years and then progress quickly, but if you are not aware of the signs to look out for, which most people that are not in the medical community aren't aware of, you don't know what started it.

Yes, individuals are going to have a tough time. Financially dysautonomia can take a toll on families. Dysautonomia can change everyday life for everyone acquainted with the patient. It affects a family's quality of life. The patient is already aware of this, they do not need to be reminded of how they are a burden to others. If you feel that you are not able to support this friend or family member, be honest. They would rather honesty then have cruelty.

If you don't know exactly what they are going through, ask them, don't just assume you know. As a patient, you need to make sure again that you advocate in a kind way. Just because you feel something on the inside, doesn't mean that it is obvious to others on the outside.

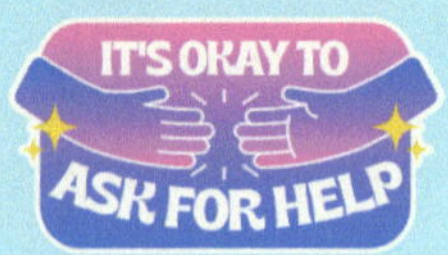

BE KIND
TO ALL
KIND

<u>Ways to manage and treat: (this is not medical advice, please consult with your doctor)</u>

Your doctor might try non-pharmacological changes to your lifestyle first.
Be patient, sometimes they can help. They do have a lower side effect risk.

Avoid certain triggers that can flair your symptoms. Keep your journal, advocate for yourself, if you start
a new medicine keep a log to notify your physician. Get sleep, practice self-care, avoid the heat, if possible,
exercise, avoid alcohol, follow the recommendations by your doctors.

There are many diets out there, especially if you have stomach issues such as IBS or IBD.
A gastroenterologist will be able to guide you on what is best for your body.

Hydration: Drink LOTS OF WATER!!! Not all in one sitting of course, spread it throughout the day.
If you can't tolerate the taste of plain water, add flavor packets such as a liquid IV or something that has
sodium, or just a flavored addition. You will want to make sure you are getting the water in!

Salt: doctors will tell you if adding additional salt to your diet is necessary.

Medications: there are many medicines out there. There are ones that help with central
nervous system stimulants, meds that help with central nervous system depressants, beta-blockers,
mineralocorticoid, central sympatholytic medications, anxiety meds, and more...... Your doctor will be able to
determine what is the best treatment approach.

It does not happen quickly though, and many trials might need to be completed before a doctor gets it right.
Doses may need to be adjusted as well, especially in growing children.

If you don't find a doctor that you connect with that understands dysautonomia, keep looking.
Ask around, families that have been through this are going to be your best resources around.
There are many social media groups that have support groups. Some have monthly virtual meetings so that
you don't have to be there in person. Sometimes it can benefit to hear from others.

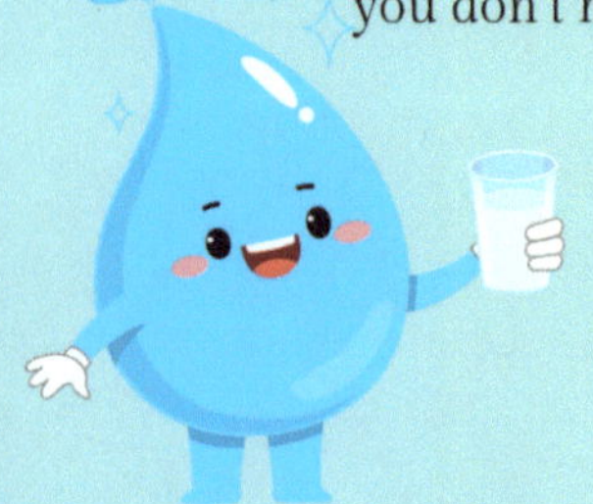

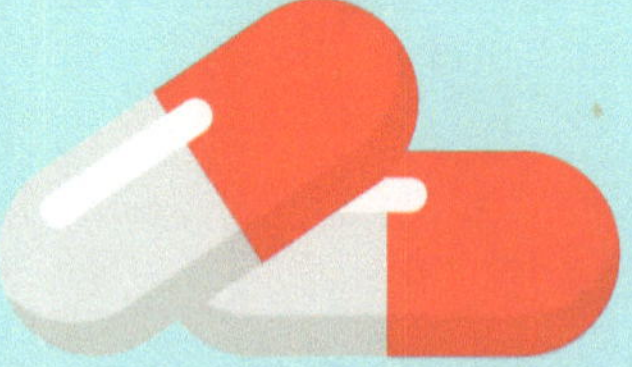

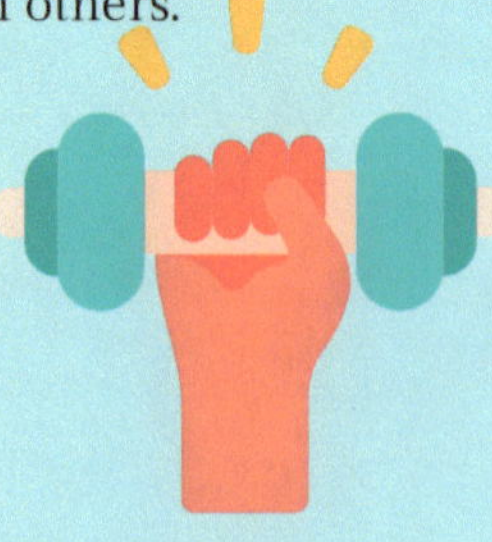

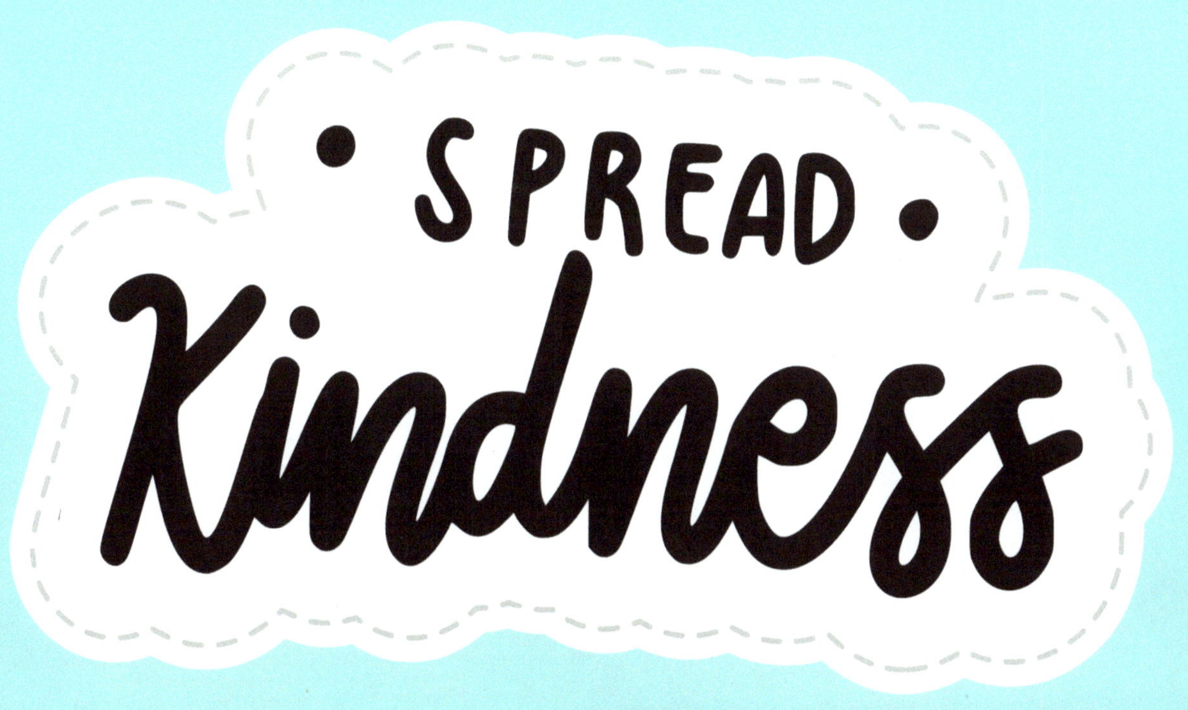

• SPREAD •
Kindness

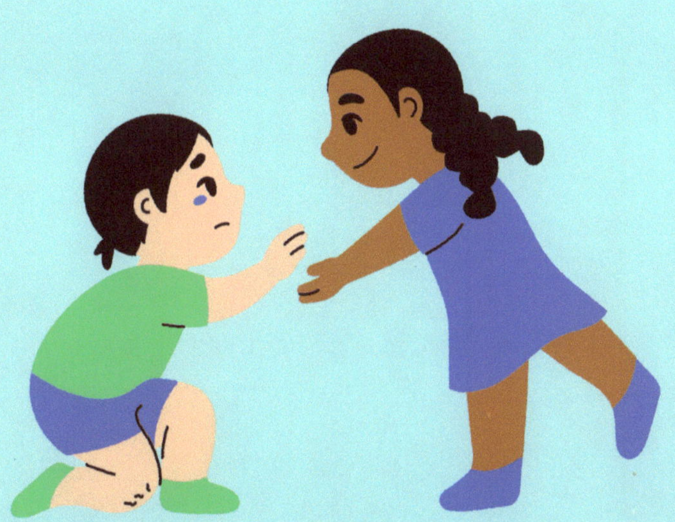

Dysautonomia Awareness Month is in October!

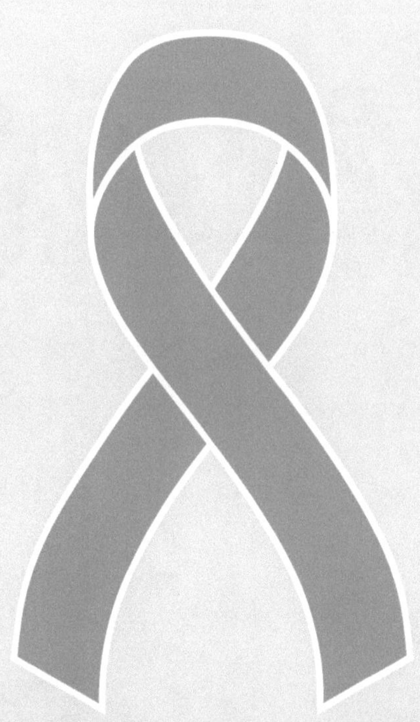

Treatment approaches are not one-size-fits-all. Just because a method worked for one person doesn't guarantee it will be the best fit for you.

Always consult with a physician before starting any treatment or program.

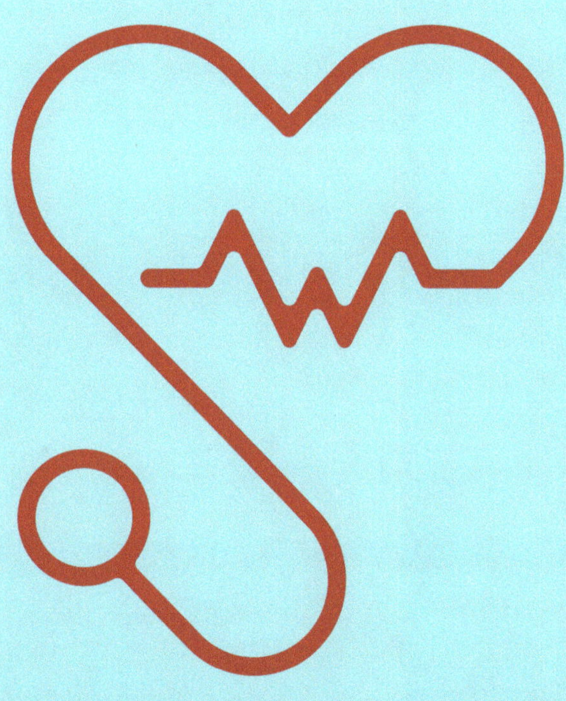

THANK YOU!!!
I want to continually thank my cousin-crew (Stephanie, Jeff, Ella Hart, Josh, Andi, Riley, Spencer and Gerald) for all of your continued love, support and patience as I continue to keep writing and researching!

You continue to amaze me with how you support our little guy as he continues to go on this journey. Riley, you are the most amazing and beautiful soul and the love and tenderness you give your brother and patience and understanding is beyond words.

Thank you for getting on the floor with us while at the beach in the middle of a gift shop and asking for fans and water, while I focused on him not passing out fully. Also, thank you for adapting vacations when it was so hot outside. Your understanding and empathy goes beyond words.

To my family and friends:
Thank you for taking the time to learn about Dysautonomia. This means a lot as we have felt very supported and not alone in this journey. This journey can be very isolating at times as no one fully understands what an individual is going through or feeling.

Thank you Gigi for understanding while on vacations that some days it was just too hot and we needed to rest. To Mema, when we would visit you and we had to adapt to his schedule for rest breaks. Both of your love, kindness, strength and support is what helps us get through.

We are truly very grateful and blessed with our village of support.

To my amazing hubby that edited the book. My ADHD brain goes awry and I definitely am thankful for you and your never ending love and support and guidance!
I am grateful that we are on this journey together and your support during doctors visits, taking notes while I am trying to absorb information and answer questions that our little guy can't always put into his own words.

Thank you to the following organizations for your continued research:

Dysautonomia International

The Dysautonomia Project

Dysautonomia Support Network

This author receives no benefits, financial or otherwise, from any of the organizations mentioned in this book.

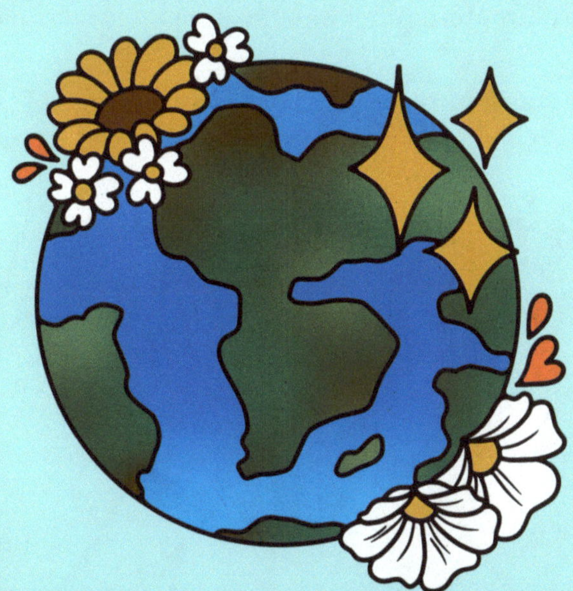

This is just a mom on a mission to help spread the word about dysautonomia and trying to save the world, one book at a time!

Thank you!

There are also many hospitals and clinics that are completing research studies as we speak.

There are many courses available online as well to watch and learn about your condition.

Research different social media groups that can be supportive when you feel alone.

It is continually changing but your life can be changed as well!

Stay strong and REACH OUT FOR HELP!

You are not alone!

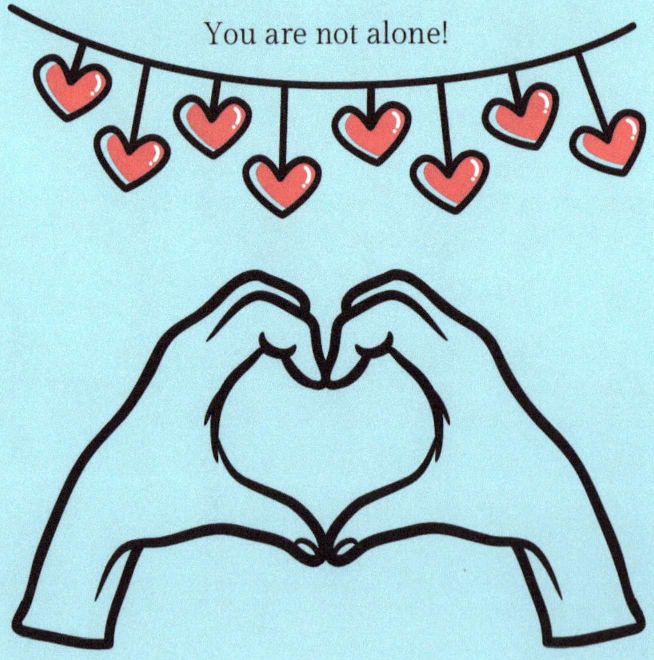

About the author:
My name is Dr. Nikki Pollack. I have been a pediatric Occupational therapist for 20 years!
I am a mom of two amazing kids and a wife to an awesome husband that is very patient
with me and my crazy ideas. I love to learn new things and am trying to find ways every day
to help others.

Whether it be researching about dysautonomia or trying to help those with frontal temporal
dementia, or just helping others in general, my love is helping individuals be their best self
in their way possible.

I graduated from the University of Alabama with my bachelor's degree, then University of St.
Augustine with my master's degree in occupational therapy. I then pursued and have
completed my doctorate in Occupational therapy from Spalding University.

I am blessed that I get to wake up every day and work with some of the most amazing kids
with different dis-ABILITIES! We don't look at what they can't do, but what they can do!
Growing up with a learning disability in math as well as with ADHD (non-combined type),
truly made me who I am today. I don't give up easily on anyone, especially when they want
their quality of life to be as great as it can be.
The reason I wrote this book, is because not everyone's journey is going to look the same and
that's okay. Don't compare yourself with others, that will get you no where except maybe
into a depressed state of mind. You are you. You rock you. If you only get out of bed today
and brush your teeth, you have done something! One day at a time, one step at a time and
remember, you are never ALONE!

Check out the Dysautonomia Journal and the
book my son wrote about his own
journey with dysautonomia.

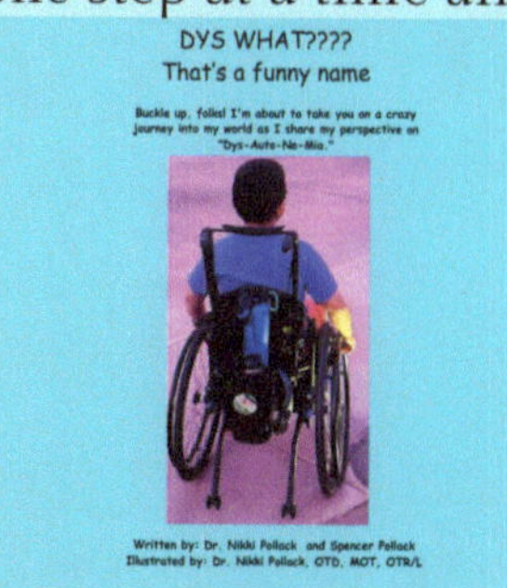